CONTEMPLATING COURAGE

MELISSA GORMAN PA-C, MPAS

CONTEMPLATING COURAGE

A REFLECTIVE JOURNALING COMPANION WHEN LIVING WITH CANCER

A guide for sharing your story.

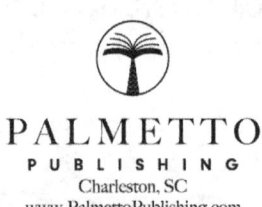

PALMETTO
PUBLISHING
Charleston, SC
www.PalmettoPublishing.com

Copyright © 2024 by Melissa Gorman PA-C, MPAS

All rights reserved

No portion of this book may be reproduced, stored in a retrieval system, or transmitted in any form by any means–electronic, mechanical, photocopy, recording, or other–except for brief quotations in printed reviews, without prior permission of the author.

Paperback ISBN: 979-8-8229-4469-5
Hardcover ISBN: 979-8-8229-5661-2

Dear Reader,

This reflective journal is written to give you a space to share your story, work through difficult decisions, and to help guide you through scenarios a cancer diagnosis may bring. It is written for those who have just been diagnosed and those who have had cancer for some time. Processing a cancer diagnosis, of any kind, can be complex and emotional. My hope is that these pages provide some degree of comfort in that process.

I am a licensed Physician Associate practicing in inpatient adult medical oncology at an academic medical center. In the hospital, I work with a specialized team to take care of people with all types of cancer, at varying stages, who require hospitalization for a myriad of conditions (directly cancer-related or not). Doing so, I have the distinct pleasure of getting to know and care for many remarkable people. They come from all walks of life, local to international, linked by one common denominator: a cancer diagnosis.

Getting to know many of my patients and their loved ones on a deeper level, often caring for them for weeks to months throughout the course of their illness, for me, has been a formative experience. Their words and lack thereof, their tears and laughter, their anger and frustration, as well as their hope. Conversations we've shared about life, death, hobbies, pets, wildest dreams and deepest fears, which protein shake the hospital cafeteria does best, when they last moved their bowels... Their stories and experiences are my motivation for writing this journal. A supportive piece of a much larger puzzle. I hope this helps you work through the sometimes monstrous-feeling battle that can be cancer.

The blessing of inpatient medical oncology is often being able to make a positive real-time difference in someone's life by controlling or treating a symptom of illness. The curse is that those who I treat and get to know at increasing frequency are likely also those who are getting sicker. Seeing as how I only work in the hospital, me seeing someone more often sadly means they are requiring more frequent hospital stays to combat infections, progressing disease, or sequelae of illness. I am often having difficult conversations with my patients and their families about what is important to them, and how to navigate roads we all hope and pray we'll never walk down. In these 'goals of care' meetings, many voiced wishing they had "thought about these things earlier," that they'd go back and do 'x' differently if they'd known 'y,' or wishing they knew how to better identify and express their wants or needs. Hence, this journal.

My goal in writing this journal is to provide you a space to share your truest thoughts. Inside, you'll find a variety of prompts ranging from your diagnosis, who you are, working with your care team, your hopes, and some more serious ones centering around end of life. Some prompts may stir up difficult feelings; give yourself grace and take this journal at whatever pace makes sense for you. Skip around. If you're struggling mentally or emotionally, I encourage you to please talk to your loved ones or seek professional help.

This journal is here to help you uncover your inner strength, explore your hopes, fears, and dreams, and just be you—fully and completely. So, let's take a journey through these pages together, where honesty and resilience meet.

Take care,
Melissa

date: grateful for:

PROUD OF	CHALLENGED BY

Write about when you were first diagnosed with cancer. Where were you? What led to your diagnosis? If it's been some time since that day, how have your feelings evolved since?

_____
_____
_____
_____
_____
_____
_____
_____
_____
_____
_____
_____
_____
_____
_____
_____
_____
_____
_____
_____
_____
_____
_____
_____

date: grateful for:

PROUD OF   **CHALLENGED BY**

What are the most significant changes you've noticed
in your daily life and routine since your diagnosis?

_____
_____
_____
_____
_____
_____
_____
_____
_____
_____
_____
_____
_____
_____
_____
_____
_____
_____
_____
_____
_____
_____
_____
_____
_____
_____

date: grateful for:

PROUD OF | **CHALLENGED BY**

Have you experienced feelings of denial or disbelief about your diagnosis? In what ways? How are you working through these feelings?

CONTEMPLATING COURAGE

date: grateful for:

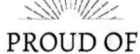

| PROUD OF | CHALLENGED BY |

In what ways has your diagnosis impacted your relationships with family and friends? How have dynamics shifted?

_____
_____
_____
_____
_____
_____
_____
_____
_____
_____
_____
_____
_____
_____
_____
_____
_____
_____
_____
_____
_____
_____
_____
_____
_____
_____

date: _____ grateful for: _____

PROUD OF	CHALLENGED BY

Prior to your cancer diagnosis, describe your relationship with the healthcare system. Are you someone who saw a clinician routinely? Only if absolutely necessary?

_____
_____
_____
_____
_____
_____
_____
_____
_____
_____
_____
_____
_____
_____
_____
_____
_____
_____
_____
_____
_____
_____
_____

date: _____   grateful for: _____

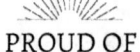

| PROUD OF | CHALLENGED BY |

Whether you've received routine medical care throughout your life or not, starting cancer treatments can often bring with it a slew of clinician visits, labs, medications, infusions, transfusions—a lot of time in and out of appointments. It can be overwhelming. How can you find, or have you found, balance?

_____
_____
_____
_____
_____
_____
_____
_____
_____
_____
_____
_____
_____
_____
_____
_____
_____
_____
_____
_____
_____
_____

date: grateful for:

PROUD OF   **CHALLENGED BY**

Who can you turn to for help if and when you need it?
Make a list of who in your life you can lean on if you need help with grocery shopping, running errands, house projects/cleaning, emotional support, childcare, etc.

_____
_____
_____
_____
_____
_____
_____
_____
_____
_____
_____
_____
_____
_____
_____
_____
_____
_____
_____
_____
_____
_____
_____
_____
_____

date: grateful for:

PROUD OF	CHALLENGED BY

Write about someone you care about and why they're important to you.
_____
_____
_____
_____
_____
_____
_____
_____
_____
_____
_____
_____
_____
_____
_____
_____
_____
_____
_____
_____
_____
_____
_____
_____
_____
_____
_____

date: grateful for:

PROUD OF | **CHALLENGED BY**

Prior to cancer, how did you handle stress?

_____
_____
_____
_____
_____
_____
_____
_____
_____
_____
_____
_____
_____
_____
_____
_____
_____
_____
_____
_____
_____
_____
_____
_____
_____
_____
_____

date: grateful for:

PROUD OF	CHALLENGED BY

What strategies do you continue to use?
What strategies have you developed for managing stress and anxiety related to your diagnosis and treatment? If you're not sure, think about some things you can implement going forward.

_____
_____
_____
_____
_____
_____
_____
_____
_____
_____
_____
_____
_____
_____
_____
_____
_____
_____
_____

date: grateful for:

PROUD OF	CHALLENGED BY

How can you help yourself navigate times of uncertainty and unpredictability?

_____
_____
_____
_____
_____
_____
_____
_____
_____
_____
_____
_____
_____
_____
_____
_____
_____
_____
_____
_____
_____
_____
_____
_____
_____

date: grateful for:

| PROUD OF | CHALLENGED BY |

What do you need from those around you to navigate times of uncertainty and unpredictability?

_____
_____
_____
_____
_____
_____
_____
_____
_____
_____
_____
_____
_____
_____
_____
_____
_____
_____
_____
_____
_____
_____

date: grateful for:

PROUD OF	CHALLENGED BY

Has your body image or self-esteem been affected by physical changes resulting from cancer or its treatments? Reflect on how you're feeling and why.

_____
_____
_____
_____
_____
_____
_____
_____
_____
_____
_____
_____
_____
_____
_____
_____
_____
_____
_____
_____
_____
_____

date: grateful for:

PROUD OF | **CHALLENGED BY**

What role does humor or laughter play in your life?

_____
_____
_____
_____
_____
_____
_____
_____
_____
_____
_____
_____
_____
_____
_____
_____
_____
_____
_____
_____
_____
_____
_____
_____
_____

date: _____ grateful for: _____

PROUD OF

CHALLENGED BY

Have you explored any support groups or counseling services to help you process your emotions or to connect with others having similar experiences? Why or why not?

_____
_____
_____
_____
_____
_____
_____
_____
_____
_____
_____
_____
_____
_____
_____
_____
_____
_____
_____
_____
_____
_____
_____
_____
_____
_____
_____

date: grateful for:

PROUD OF	CHALLENGED BY

If you could switch lives with anyone for a day, who would it be and why?

date: _____   grateful for: _____

PROUD OF	CHALLENGED BY

What has been the most challenging aspect of your cancer journey so far? How have you attempted to overcome it?

_____
_____
_____
_____
_____
_____
_____
_____
_____
_____
_____
_____
_____
_____
_____
_____
_____
_____
_____
_____
_____
_____
_____
_____
_____
_____
_____

date: grateful for:

PROUD OF   CHALLENGED BY

Are there specific goals or milestones you've set for yourself during your cancer treatment? How do you track your progress?

_____
_____
_____
_____
_____
_____
_____
_____
_____
_____
_____
_____
_____
_____
_____
_____
_____
_____
_____
_____
_____
_____
_____

date: grateful for:

PROUD OF | **CHALLENGED BY**

What is something you wish you could tell
your younger, or childhood, self and why?

_____
_____
_____
_____
_____
_____
_____
_____
_____
_____
_____
_____
_____
_____
_____
_____
_____
_____
_____
_____
_____
_____
_____
_____
_____
_____

date: grateful for:

PROUD OF	CHALLENGED BY

How has your relationship with yourself, your body, and your mortality evolved since your diagnosis?

_____
_____
_____
_____
_____
_____
_____
_____
_____
_____
_____
_____
_____
_____
_____
_____
_____
_____
_____
_____
_____
_____
_____
_____

date: grateful for:

PROUD OF | **CHALLENGED BY**

What are your personal beliefs about the role of mind-body connections in healing or times of stress or unease? How can you incorporate mindfulness into your life?

_____
_____
_____
_____
_____
_____
_____
_____
_____
_____
_____
_____
_____
_____
_____
_____
_____
_____
_____
_____
_____
_____
_____
_____
_____
_____

date: grateful for:

PROUD OF	CHALLENGED BY

How do you handle conversations about your cancer with people who may not understand your experience or may unintentionally say hurtful things?

_____
_____
_____
_____
_____
_____
_____
_____
_____
_____
_____
_____
_____
_____
_____
_____
_____
_____
_____
_____

date: grateful for:

| PROUD OF | CHALLENGED BY |

How do you make decisions about treatment options and medical procedures? What factors are most important to you in those decisions?

_____
_____
_____
_____
_____
_____
_____
_____
_____
_____
_____
_____
_____
_____
_____
_____
_____
_____
_____
_____
_____
_____
_____
_____
_____
_____

date:	grateful for:
PROUD OF	CHALLENGED BY

How do you best learn and receive information?
Are you a visual learner where pictures and figures are most helpful?
Do you learn best by listening? By doing? By writing and repeating?
Does your cancer team know your preference?

_____
_____
_____
_____
_____
_____
_____
_____
_____
_____
_____
_____
_____
_____
_____
_____
_____
_____
_____
_____
_____
_____

date: grateful for:

PROUD OF | **CHALLENGED BY**

What do you hope for?

date: grateful for:

PROUD OF	CHALLENGED BY

In what way(s) has your perspective on life changed because of your cancer diagnosis?

_____
_____
_____
_____
_____
_____
_____
_____
_____
_____
_____
_____
_____
_____
_____
_____
_____
_____
_____
_____
_____

date: _____   grateful for: _____

PROUD OF	CHALLENGED BY

Make a list of the people and things that bring you joy.

_____
_____
_____
_____
_____
_____
_____
_____
_____
_____
_____
_____
_____
_____
_____
_____
_____
_____
_____
_____
_____
_____
_____
_____
_____
_____
_____
_____
_____

date: grateful for:

PROUD OF | **CHALLENGED BY**

Make a list of words and phrases
that your friends or family would use to describe you.

date: grateful for:

PROUD OF	CHALLENGED BY

What scares you?

_____
_____
_____
_____
_____
_____
_____
_____
_____
_____
_____
_____
_____
_____
_____
_____
_____
_____
_____
_____
_____
_____
_____
_____
_____
_____

date: grateful for:

PROUD OF	CHALLENGED BY

What coping strategies have you found most effective in managing the emotional aspects of cancer? If you feel like you haven't been coping in ways you'd like, what can you do about that?
Brainstorm ways you could healthily cope and process your feelings.

_____
_____
_____
_____
_____
_____
_____
_____
_____
_____
_____
_____
_____
_____
_____
_____
_____
_____
_____
_____
_____
_____

date: grateful for:

PROUD OF | **CHALLENGED BY**

Describe your relationship with your healthcare team.
How has it evolved over time?

_____
_____
_____
_____
_____
_____
_____
_____
_____
_____
_____
_____
_____
_____
_____
_____
_____
_____
_____
_____
_____
_____

date: grateful for:

PROUD OF	CHALLENGED BY

Are there any unexpected positive aspects or personal growth that you've experienced as a result of your cancer journey? Things you've come to know better about yourself?

_____
_____
_____
_____
_____
_____
_____
_____
_____
_____
_____
_____
_____
_____
_____
_____
_____
_____
_____
_____
_____
_____
_____

date: _____   grateful for: _____

PROUD OF	CHALLENGED BY

What motivates you?

_____
_____
_____
_____
_____
_____
_____
_____
_____
_____
_____
_____
_____
_____
_____
_____
_____
_____
_____
_____
_____
_____
_____
_____
_____
_____
_____
_____
_____

date: grateful for:

PROUD OF	CHALLENGED BY

Prior to your cancer diagnosis, describe your communication style. How do you communicate with those close to you? With co-workers? With strangers?

_____
_____
_____
_____
_____
_____
_____
_____
_____
_____
_____
_____
_____
_____
_____
_____
_____
_____
_____
_____
_____
_____
_____

date: grateful for:

PROUD OF | **CHALLENGED BY**

How do you communicate with your loved ones about your cancer? How has this communication evolved?

date: grateful for:

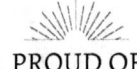

PROUD OF | CHALLENGED BY

This one is for all the internalizers out there. Do you feel you are able to communicate openly with your loved ones or do you feel like you bury your feelings, dismiss them, or keep everything in?
My hope is you will find at least one person in your life (personally or professionally like a therapist) who you can open up to. I challenge you to talk about your hopes, fears, and wishes. Cancer is difficult. Internalizing all that you're going through can feel isolating and you deserve to be heard, validated, and feel cared for emotionally.
I respectfully encourage you to reflect here about why you may find difficulty in opening up and expressing emotion to others.

date:	grateful for:
PROUD OF	CHALLENGED BY

If you have children, young or grown, how do you communicate with your children about your cancer and how you are feeling? Do you hold information back? If so, why? Do you need guidance on age-friendly ways to talk about cancer, the good and the bad?

_____
_____
_____
_____
_____
_____
_____
_____
_____
_____
_____
_____
_____
_____
_____
_____
_____
_____
_____
_____

date: grateful for:

PROUD OF | **CHALLENGED BY**

Cancer aside, what do you want your children to know and understand about you as a person?

_____
_____
_____
_____
_____
_____
_____
_____
_____
_____
_____
_____
_____
_____
_____
_____
_____
_____
_____
_____
_____
_____
_____
_____
_____
_____

date: grateful for:

PROUD OF | **CHALLENGED BY**

Write about some of your favorite things about yourself.

date: grateful for:

| PROUD OF | CHALLENGED BY |

Write about your proudest accomplishment.

date:	grateful for:
PROUD OF	CHALLENGED BY

How can you facilitate open and honest conversations with your family about your needs and desires? Are there ways your loved ones can better support you in your cancer journey that you haven't yet shared with them? Friendly reminder, they cannot read your mind.

date: grateful for:

PROUD OF   ## CHALLENGED BY

What strategies do you use to manage side effects from treatments?

date: grateful for:

PROUD OF	CHALLENGED BY

Which symptoms do you manage well?
Which symptoms do you feel are poorly controlled?

_____
_____
_____
_____
_____
_____
_____
_____
_____
_____
_____
_____
_____
_____
_____
_____
_____
_____
_____
_____
_____
_____
_____
_____

date: _____   grateful for: _____

PROUD OF	**CHALLENGED BY**

How can you talk to your care team about your symptoms that are poorly controlled? What are your expectations? What are you able to tolerate in terms of your symptoms (i.e., pain, etc) and what needs some work?

_____
_____
_____
_____
_____
_____
_____
_____
_____
_____
_____
_____
_____
_____
_____
_____
_____
_____
_____
_____
_____
_____
_____
_____

CONTEMPLATING COURAGE

date: grateful for:

PROUD OF	CHALLENGED BY

How do you find moments of joy and gratitude during challenging times?

_____
_____
_____
_____
_____
_____
_____
_____
_____
_____
_____
_____
_____
_____
_____
_____
_____
_____
_____
_____
_____
_____
_____
_____

date: grateful for:

PROUD OF   **CHALLENGED BY**

What resources have been most valuable to you?
What could you use additional information about?

date: grateful for:

PROUD OF 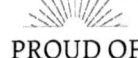	CHALLENGED BY

Malnutrition is a common problem for people with cancer. Significant weight loss often compounded by nausea, vomiting, poor appetite... what are ways you find helpful to combat malnutrition? If you're struggling with eating, how might you increase your calorie and protein intake?

_____
_____
_____
_____
_____
_____
_____
_____
_____
_____
_____
_____
_____
_____
_____
_____
_____
_____
_____

date: grateful for:

PROUD OF	CHALLENGED BY

If there became a point where you were having difficulty maintaining adequate nutrition on your own, would you want a temporary feeding tube in your nose, or a long-term/permanent feeding tube in your stomach if deemed feasible and medically appropriate for you?

_____
_____
_____
_____
_____
_____
_____
_____
_____
_____
_____
_____
_____
_____
_____
_____
_____
_____
_____
_____
_____

date: grateful for:

PROUD OF	CHALLENGED BY

Think about a moment when you felt completely content and at peace. Write about it here. What were you doing? Where were you? Were you with anyone else?

_____
_____
_____
_____
_____
_____
_____
_____
_____
_____
_____
_____
_____
_____
_____
_____
_____
_____
_____
_____
_____
_____
_____
_____

date: grateful for:

PROUD OF | **CHALLENGED BY**

Do you have the support you need? If so, describe what that looks like. If you don't, brainstorm ways you can build it.

_____
_____
_____
_____
_____
_____
_____
_____
_____
_____
_____
_____
_____
_____
_____
_____
_____
_____
_____
_____
_____
_____
_____
_____

date: grateful for:

PROUD OF   **CHALLENGED BY**

Make a list of 5 things about your body you are grateful for.

date: grateful for:

PROUD OF	CHALLENGED BY

Who or what inspires you?

date: grateful for:

PROUD OF | **CHALLENGED BY**

How do you handle uncertainty about the future?

date: grateful for:

PROUD OF   **CHALLENGED BY**

Write about a time when you felt like you were able to make a positive difference in someone else's life.

CONTEMPLATING COURAGE

date: grateful for:

PROUD OF | **CHALLENGED BY**

Write down three affirmations that reinforce your value and self-worth.

date: grateful for:

PROUD OF	CHALLENGED BY

Think back on a milestone or celebratory event that sticks out to you and makes you smile. Write about it and why it was so special.

_____
_____
_____
_____
_____
_____
_____
_____
_____
_____
_____
_____
_____
_____
_____
_____
_____
_____
_____
_____
_____
_____
_____
_____
_____

date: grateful for:

PROUD OF | CHALLENGED BY

Has your oncologist discussed your prognosis and if the goal of your cancer treatment is of curative intent (goal is cancer free) or palliative intent (goal is to slow cancer growth and treat symptoms, but is not curable)? Is this something important to you? How does knowing or not knowing cause you to live and plan differently?

_____
_____
_____
_____
_____
_____
_____
_____
_____
_____
_____
_____
_____
_____
_____
_____
_____
_____
_____
_____

date: grateful for:

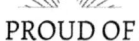
PROUD OF   CHALLENGED BY

Are there any lifestyle changes or habits you've adopted to support your overall well-being? Give yourself grace and credit if you have—new habits can be hard to form. Write about new habits you've formed and how you did, or habits you hope to form and how to do so.

_____
_____
_____
_____
_____
_____
_____
_____
_____
_____
_____
_____
_____
_____
_____
_____
_____
_____
_____
_____
_____

date: grateful for:

PROUD OF | **CHALLENGED BY**

Write about a time you felt isolated or disconnected from those around you. Write about what that felt like. What might you do to feel more connected?

date: grateful for:

PROUD OF	CHALLENGED BY

Reflect on a time you felt truly loved and supported.
Describe what that felt like and its impact on you.

_____
_____
_____
_____
_____
_____
_____
_____
_____
_____
_____
_____
_____
_____
_____
_____
_____
_____
_____
_____
_____
_____
_____

date: grateful for:

PROUD OF | **CHALLENGED BY**

What lessons have you learned about resilience and strength through your experience with cancer?

___

date: _____ grateful for: _____

| PROUD OF | CHALLENGED BY |

How has your sense of purpose evolved since your cancer diagnosis? How have your life goals changed? What new priorities have emerged?

_____
_____
_____
_____
_____
_____
_____
_____
_____
_____
_____
_____
_____
_____
_____
_____
_____
_____
_____
_____
_____
_____
_____
_____
_____
_____

date: grateful for:

PROUD OF | CHALLENGED BY

Have you explored complementary therapies or alternative cancer treatments? If so, what has been your experience with them?

date:	grateful for:
PROUD OF	CHALLENGED BY

What do you need right now?

_____
_____
_____
_____
_____
_____
_____
_____
_____
_____
_____
_____
_____
_____
_____
_____
_____
_____
_____
_____
_____
_____
_____
_____
_____

date: grateful for:

PROUD OF | CHALLENGED BY

What are your short-term goals?

_____
_____
_____
_____
_____
_____
_____
_____
_____
_____
_____
_____
_____
_____
_____
_____
_____
_____
_____
_____
_____
_____
_____
_____
_____
_____
_____

date: grateful for:

PROUD OF	CHALLENGED BY

What brings you happiness right now? This can be people in your life, intangible things, hobbies... anything!

_____
_____
_____
_____
_____
_____
_____
_____
_____
_____
_____
_____
_____
_____
_____
_____
_____
_____
_____
_____
_____
_____
_____
_____
_____

date: grateful for:

| PROUD OF | CHALLENGED BY |

Reflect on the role that spirituality or faith plays in your life, if at all.
Is spirituality or faith something that has always been part of your life?
Do you want it to be?

date: _____ grateful for: _____

PROUD OF

CHALLENGED BY

How do you balance taking care of your physical health with your emotional and mental well-being?

_____
_____
_____
_____
_____
_____
_____
_____
_____
_____
_____
_____
_____
_____
_____
_____
_____
_____
_____
_____
_____
_____
_____
_____

date:	grateful for:
PROUD OF	**CHALLENGED BY**

What advice would you give to someone newly diagnosed with cancer based on your own experiences?

_____
_____
_____
_____
_____
_____
_____
_____
_____
_____
_____
_____
_____
_____
_____
_____
_____
_____
_____
_____
_____
_____
_____
_____
_____

date: grateful for:

PROUD OF | **CHALLENGED BY**

What are your greatest hopes and aspirations moving forward?

_____
_____
_____
_____
_____
_____
_____
_____
_____
_____
_____
_____
_____
_____
_____
_____
_____
_____
_____
_____
_____
_____
_____
_____
_____
_____
_____

date: grateful for:

PROUD OF	CHALLENGED BY

What does 'quality of life' mean to you?
What does good quality of life look like for you?

_____
_____
_____
_____
_____
_____
_____
_____
_____
_____
_____
_____
_____
_____
_____
_____
_____
_____
_____
_____
_____
_____
_____
_____
_____

date: grateful for:

PROUD OF

CHALLENGED BY

Reflecting on your journey with cancer, consider this: If given the choice, would you prioritize *quality* of life: cherishing each moment with whatever functionality you have, even if it means a shorter time or stopping treatments? OR. Would you opt for a longer *quantity* of time, even if it comes with more challenges like hospital time, drug side effects, less stamina/ functionality, or makes you sicker? Which aspects of your life bring you the most joy, fulfillment, and peace? How do these factors influence your choice between *quality* and *quantity* in the face of cancer?

_____
_____
_____
_____
_____
_____
_____
_____
_____
_____
_____
_____
_____
_____
_____
_____
_____
_____
_____

date: grateful for:

PROUD OF | **CHALLENGED BY**

Write about any specific milestones or experiences you hope to achieve in the time ahead?

date: _____   grateful for: _____

PROUD OF

CHALLENGED BY

Do you have a healthcare Power of Attorney document? If you do, write about who you designated. What do they mean to you? If you don't, brainstorm who you would name (typically two people a 1st and 2nd) to make medical decisions on your behalf if you are deemed medically unable to do so. Contact your medical team about creating this document.

_____
_____
_____
_____
_____
_____
_____
_____
_____
_____
_____
_____
_____
_____
_____
_____
_____
_____
_____
_____
_____

date: grateful for:

PROUD OF   **CHALLENGED BY**

If you are facing a terminal diagnosis, how do you hope to align your medical treatment and personal goals to make the most of whatever time you have left?

___

date: grateful for:

PROUD OF   **CHALLENGED BY**

What are your most intrusive fears or worries
regarding your cancer diagnosis or what is to come?

_____
_____
_____
_____
_____
_____
_____
_____
_____
_____
_____
_____
_____
_____
_____
_____
_____
_____
_____
_____
_____
_____
_____
_____
_____
_____

date:　　　　　　　　　　　grateful for:

| PROUD OF | CHALLENGED BY |

How do these fears affect your daily life and decision-making?

date: grateful for:

PROUD OF | **CHALLENGED BY**

What steps can you take to find moments of peace and relief from your fears?

date:　　　　　　　　　　grateful for:

PROUD OF　　　　　　**CHALLENGED BY**

How can you communicate your fears and concerns with your healthcare team? How do you hope they will support you? How can you ask for what you need?

_____
_____
_____
_____
_____
_____
_____
_____
_____
_____
_____
_____
_____
_____
_____
_____
_____
_____
_____
_____
_____
_____
_____

date: grateful for:

PROUD OF | **CHALLENGED BY**

How can you communicate your fears and concerns with your loved ones?

date: grateful for:

PROUD OF

CHALLENGED BY

What would you like your loved ones to better understand about your experience with cancer?

_____
_____
_____
_____
_____
_____
_____
_____
_____
_____
_____
_____
_____
_____
_____
_____
_____
_____
_____
_____
_____
_____
_____
_____

date: grateful for:

PROUD OF | **CHALLENGED BY**

Are there specific things you want to communicate to your loved ones but find challenging to express? Explore why they are challenging.

_____
_____
_____
_____
_____
_____
_____
_____
_____
_____
_____
_____
_____
_____
_____
_____
_____
_____
_____
_____
_____
_____
_____
_____
_____
_____
_____

date: grateful for:

PROUD OF	CHALLENGED BY

Reflect on a recent moment that brought you comfort or joy.
What made it special?

___

date: grateful for:

PROUD OF   **CHALLENGED BY**

How can you incorporate more moments that bring joy into your life?
___

date: grateful for:

PROUD OF	CHALLENGED BY

Explore moments when you've been hard on yourself during this journey. How can you practice self-compassion and treat yourself with the same kindness you would offer a friend facing similar challenges?

_____
_____
_____
_____
_____
_____
_____
_____
_____
_____
_____
_____
_____
_____
_____
_____
_____
_____
_____
_____
_____
_____
_____

date: _____ grateful for: _____

PROUD OF | **CHALLENGED BY**

The word "hospice" can provoke a myriad of thoughts and emotions. What does the word "hospice" mean to you? What is your understanding of hospice care? On the next page you will find more information about hospice care, but first share your impressions.

What is Hospice Care?

Generally speaking, someone becomes eligible for hospice care if they have a terminal illness, and their expected prognosis (life expectancy) is six months or less. As a general philosophy, hospice focuses on the comfort, care, and quality of life of a person with terminal illness. Hospice is not a program that aims to shorten whatever time one has left or to hasten death. The goal is comfort, resources, and symptom control to give someone quality time for whatever amount of time they have left.

Cancer is a diagnosis many of us think about when talking about hospice care, but there are several conditions like advanced heart or lung disease, kidney or liver failure, dementia, or Parkinson's that at a certain stage may qualify someone for hospice care. When it comes to a cancer diagnosis, hospice is generally recommended as a plan of care when your team worries that you have months or less to live. Hospice may become a conversation because the cancer is no longer responding to treatments, there are no more treatment options available, or there are no more viable treatment options that can be safely given due to significant risk of harm in one's particular situation. On a hospice plan of care, cancer-directed treatments are stopped and the focus shifts to caring for the person and their symptoms, not the cancer itself.

The focus becomes about symptom management and quality of life. Symptoms and care are managed by a hospice team. The hospice team is typically made up of provider(s)/a medical director, nurses, aides, social workers, spiritual services representatives, and volunteers. This grouping of people help to support patient and family, providing guidance on how to best treat symptoms as they come or change. Symptoms that hospice teams typically help to treat in end of life include but are not limited to pain, shortness of breath, anxiety, restlessness/agitation, dry mouth or eyes, nausea, and constipation. Hospice care is generally part of one's health insurance plan and tends to also cover certain medical equipment that may be needed at end of life such as a hospital bed, bedside commode, etc.

If hospice services are something you want to know more about, whether you are looking to transition to this plan of care or just looking for more information, you should talk with your oncology team. Your team can answer questions you might have and provide resources for hospice organizations that service your geographic area. If multiple organizations exist, your care team may be able to help you select one that fits your needs. Alternatively, you can arrange an informational meeting with the agency to talk about what care would look like.

Clarifications About Hospice Care

1. **Hospice is for people with terminal illness.** Hospice provides symptom management for people with serious illness, no matter their age, culture, or beliefs. As stated before, there are several end-stage conditions that qualify someone for hospice care, not just cancer.

2. **Hospice plans can be reversed.** People choose to be on hospice care and have to sign on with an agency, or if incapacitated, their healthcare power of attorney can sign onto hospice care. You can come off of hospice at any time, reversing the care plan. You can also decide to sign back onto hospice at a later date, assuming you still qualify.

3. **Hospice supports symptoms.** The hospice care team can administer medications and provide guidance to family/friends on how to administer medications to treat symptoms like pain, shortness of breath, nausea, constipation, anxiety, and more.

4. **Hospice does not shorten life.** The goal of the hospice team is to provide medicines and services that help maximize quality of life and minimize symptoms without shortening whatever time remains. The goal of hospice care is not to hasten the dying process but to allow individuals to live comfortably for however long they have.

5. **There is no expiration date for hospice care plans.** Like I talked about before, someone qualifies for hospice care when they are estimated to have six months or less to live. People are not dropped from hospice care at the six-month mark if they are still living. A hospice organization can discuss further information and policies.

6. **Hospice meets people where their condition is.** Some people are signing onto hospice care in their final moments and may only have hours to short days left, whereas some people sign onto hospice care when they have several months to live. As you might imagine, these scenarios may look quite different. For someone with 4 months to live who is moving around well and has minimal/no symptoms, the hospice team may check-in as infrequently as the person prefers, not even once per week. For someone with hours to short days to live, the hospice team is checking in far more often, making medication adjustments, offering support, etc. You are not confined to a hospital bed if you don't need to be. The hospice team wants you to be able to do things you love as long as you are able to.

7. **Hospice care can happen in various settings.** The 3 primary settings for hospice care are 1) at home, 2) a nursing home, or 3) a residential hospice facility (designated hospice hospital so to speak). Your healthcare team, social worker/case manager, or hospice liaison can help you figure out which would be best for your situation. Sometimes, certain settings are not an option depending on your needs, but the goal is for hospice care to happen where you feel comfortable and are able to be surrounded by people and things you love.

8. **You can generally keep taking some of your other medications.** For example, someone with cancer is given an estimated 4–6 months to live. This person also has asthma, has been prescribed inhalers for years, and would benefit from continuing them. Their asthma medication can continue because it is improving their quality of life, assisting with symptom management. Your team may recommend stopping medicines that have little to no benefit to you in the short-term. The hope is to cut down on non-beneficial medications that just add to your overall "pill

burden" or the number of pills you must take. Your team can help give recommendations for your specific situation.

9. **With home hospice, family and friends are the primary caregivers**. On a home hospice care plan, family and friends are the primary caregivers 24/7 and are responsible for general cares and administering medicines. Generally, the hospice team will visit and check-in to help family, do assessments, and make adjustments but likely only for 1–2 hours up to a few times per week. Family may opt to hire private caregivers or assistance at home if financially feasible. Talk to your local hospice agency about any questions you may have.

10. **With home hospice, insurance generally covers equipment you may need**. When people elect to do hospice at home, their hospice insurance benefit usually covers equipment needed at home to ease suffering and promote quality of life. This may include a hospital bed, toileting support like a bedside commode, shower chair, oxygen tank, etc. Please check with your insurance provider to be sure, or if you have a case manager/social worker they may be able to assist you with finding this information.

11. **With residential hospice, or nursing homes with hospice, there may be a room and board cost**. In certain scenarios, there can be "room and board" fees associated with being in a facility and receiving hospice care. Whether there is a fee may depend on someone's qualifying symptom needs or overall prognosis. This fee is entirely separate from the hospice-related services themselves, which are generally covered by insurance under the hospice benefit. You should talk to your care team, hospice agency liaison, or social worker/case manager about hospice settings and possible associated costs.

12. **Generally, those on hospice don't have out of pocket costs *for hospice-related services*.** Medicare covers up to 100% of hospice care costs for people eligible for hospice. Medicaid benefits vary by state, reach out to your care team for direction about exploring these benefits. Those on private insurance should check with their insurance provider for specifics about their hospice benefit.

13. **Hospice supports family too.** During end of life and after a loved one passes, hospice can help family with the emotional pain associated with loss. Hospice agencies generally have social workers, volunteers, and spiritual support services. They can also help connect family to support groups. Reach out to your local hospice agency or liaison about family services offered.

date: grateful for:

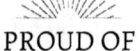
PROUD OF

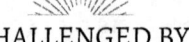
CHALLENGED BY

Have you had any discussions with your healthcare team about hospice care, and if so, how do you feel about those conversations?

date: _____   grateful for: _____

PROUD OF

CHALLENGED BY

How do you envision the role of hospice care in your journey, and what are your expectations for it? What questions or concerns do you have that you'd like to explore further?

_____
_____
_____
_____
_____
_____
_____
_____
_____
_____
_____
_____
_____
_____
_____
_____
_____
_____
_____
_____
_____
_____
_____
_____
_____

date:	grateful for:
PROUD OF	CHALLENGED BY

Write about a favorite place you've visited or experienced.

date: grateful for:

PROUD OF   CHALLENGED BY

What are your personal goals or preferences regarding end-of-life care? How can these be communicated to your healthcare team and loved ones? For example, would you rather have better pain control even if it means being more drowsy/sedated *or* would you prefer to tolerate more pain if doing so means you're more alert and able to interact more with loved ones?

_____
_____
_____
_____
_____
_____
_____
_____
_____
_____
_____
_____
_____
_____
_____
_____
_____
_____
_____
_____

Code Status Discussion

Full Code vs. DNR

Here, we will talk about code status. This information can be heavy. It is not meant to scare you but to provide background information to help you make an informed decision for yourself in your unique situation.

Code status refers to how medical personnel would respond if your heart stopped beating and you stopped breathing, meaning you have died. Naming a code status is an easy decision for some, but for many people this is a difficult conversation to have as well as a difficult decision to make and to think about.

Would you want to have chest compressions and a tube down your throat (CPR), being hooked up to a breathing machine to attempt resuscitation trying to bring you back to life? This is called being a "**Full Code**."

Alternatively, do you believe that if it's your time you would want someone to ensure you're comfortable but not attempt reviving you and not put you on a breathing machine (a ventilator). This is called being a "**Do Not Resuscitate**," or "**DNR**."

In my clinical practice as a hospital-based medical oncology provider, I have noticed some common misconceptions or misinformation expressed by patients or their families regarding what specific code status decisions mean and what they may look like in execution. Here are some clarifications that I hope will help you in your decision-making:

> Being a "DNR" or "Do Not Resuscitate" does not impact your ability to get cancer treatments, IV fluids, antibiotics, imaging/scans, any cares, placement in a rehab/nursing home/assisted living, physical therapy, etc. The only time a DNR comes into play is in the event your heart

stops beating or if you stop breathing. In that particular setting, a DNR tells your care team or emergency medical services that you wish to remain comfortable without artificial resuscitation attempts to bring you back to life. That you have passed away and it was your time; passed naturally as some would say.

Being a "Full Code" means that in those same circumstances, you want to try and be revived by cardiopulmonary resuscitation (aka CPR) which is doing chest compressions, possible defibrillation (aka electrical shock), giving medications, and inserting an artificial airway down your throat (or if unable, by procedure creating an artificial airway in your neck) to help the medical team breathe for you (usually either by a machine i.e., a ventilator or a balloon device the team can squeeze). The goal being to restart your heart and/or restore breathing.

Hollywood portrays CPR in many movies and medical TV shows as a way to revive someone quickly and easily. While sometimes true, unfortunately, that is often not the case. I have heard people cite a fear of giving up or a fear of dying as wanting CPR and choosing to be a "Full Code" but that same person also expressing not wanting to be kept alive on a breathing machine. I urge you to educate yourself further on code status nuances to best align with your goals but also with your situation. CPR is not a fail-safe intervention, but it absolutely can and does work in many scenarios. There is more information that may help you on the next page. Please talk with your healthcare team who knows you best.

What impacts how effective CPR can be?

There are many factors that play a role in the probability that CPR can resuscitate someone. Some of these include a person's age, physical stamina/condition, how quickly they are found unresponsive, if CPR is started by a trained professional, and if CPR is initiated in the hospital or out in the community. Unfortunately, advanced cancer, especially when widespread in the bones and organs makes resuscitation attempts quite difficult and oftentimes, regrettably, futile. Studies demonstrated that people with metastatic cancer had about a 9.5% chance of successful resuscitation from CPR attempts. In one meta-analysis, people with metastatic cancer who received in-hospital CPR only had a 5.6% chance of survival to discharge. CPR success rates unfortunately can diminish further if someone also has heart disease, advanced lung or other organ disease (like kidney or liver), diabetes, stroke, bowel perforation, major infection, or dementia.

What risks are associated with CPR?

Like any intervention, CPR has risks and benefits. The most hopeful benefit we can gain from CPR is successfully resuscitating someone and bringing them back to life in the same functional state they were in before the sentinel event occurred. Risks of CPR attempts include breaking ribs or other bones, damage to internal organs either by puncture or other processes, internal bleeding (at even increased risk if the person has low platelets), decreased or obsolete functional status, aspiration, or hypoxic brain damage resulting in a vegetative state.

Discussions about code status can, very understandably, raise a lot of questions. Everyone's situation is unique and individual, as is their code status choice. I advise that you talk to your medical team for further discussion and guidance if you are struggling with this. Broadly and in summary, the options for code status are as follows:

1. Full Code: try to resuscitate by doing chest compressions, possible defibrillation, giving medications, and inserting an artificial airway (or by procedure creating an artificial airway) to help the medical team breathe for you to try and restart your heart and/or restore breathing.
    or
2. Do Not Resuscitate (DNR): keep (or make) you comfortable and do not try to resuscitate, allowing for a natural death.

Whichever choice you make is absolutely yours and know that code status decisions can be reversed in either direction—if your wishes change, make sure to alert your medical care team.

date: grateful for:

PROUD OF	CHALLENGED BY

If you know your wishes about code status, here is a space to write about them. If thinking about code status brings up questions you want to ask your care team, jot those down. Otherwise, leave this blank to maybe re-visit another time.

_____
_____
_____
_____
_____
_____
_____
_____
_____
_____
_____
_____
_____
_____
_____
_____
_____
_____
_____
_____

date: grateful for:

PROUD OF	CHALLENGED BY

What legacy or message would you like to leave for your loved ones?

_____
_____
_____
_____
_____
_____
_____
_____
_____
_____
_____
_____
_____
_____
_____
_____
_____
_____
_____
_____
_____
_____
_____
_____

date: grateful for:

PROUD OF   **CHALLENGED BY**

Think of all that you've done in your life,
make a list of things you are proud of.

Wherever you are in life, my sincerest hope is
that this journal provided you with a space to reflect, grow, grieve,
reminisce, smile, and be nothing short of *you*.

This journal is dedicated to my patients and their families. To those still with us and those who have passed. Your impact on my life has been, and continues to be, profound. I could not be more grateful for the opportunity to walk alongside you as best I could. To hear your stories. To laugh and sometimes cry together. To try and make some piece of your day a little bit easier. Thank you.

About the Author

Melissa Gorman PA-C, MPAS is a physician associate currently practicing in inpatient medical oncology at an academic medical center in Milwaukee, WI. Melissa received both her bachelor's degree in biomedical science and her master's degree in PA studies from Marquette University. Outside of work, Melissa loves spending quality time with others. Her boyfriend, family (including their sweet little dog Sammy), and friends are her world. She enjoys cooking, travel, game nights, going for walks, a good book, and a crafty project. You can also find her watching college basketball (Go Marquette!!) or enjoying Kopps Custard.

At the core of Melissa's practice is a commitment to try and better understand her patients' needs, fostering meaningful connections with them as she helps navigate diagnoses and treatment plans.

A special thanks to my parents, brother, boyfriend Jon, and friends Alexis, Kim, and Tori for helping me turn this passion project into print. Here's to hoping its pages are a help to someone somewhere.

www.ingramcontent.com/pod-product-compliance
Lightning Source LLC
LaVergne TN
LVHW012053070526
838201LV00083B/4512